BIOFEEDBACK TRAINING FOR STRESS REDUCTION AND RELAXATION

Unlock Your Inner Calm with Simple Techniques to Harness the Power of Biofeedback for a Stress-Free and Relaxed Life"

DR. CHRIS FRIEDRICH

Disclaimer

This book on Herbal Remedies is intended solely for informational and educational purposes.

The content provided within this book is based on general knowledge and should not be considered as professional advice. The author is not a licensed medical professional, and the information presented here is not intended to diagnose, treat, cure, or prevent any disease.

Readers are advised to consult with qualified healthcare professionals before initiating any herbal remedies or making changes to their existing health regimen. The author and publisher disclaim any responsibility for any adverse effects or consequences resulting from the use of information contained in this book.

It's important to note that the content of this book is not endorsed by any specific platform or affiliated with any product or service.

The author does not receive any compensation or benefits from the promotion of specific herbal products or brands.

Readers should exercise their discretion and judgment when applying the information from this book, and they are encouraged to conduct further research and seek guidance from healthcare professionals to make informed decisions about their health and well-being.

"Biofeedback Training for Stress" is a thorough manual that explores the complex relationship between stress and biofeedback and provides a sophisticated look at stress management with innovative methods. The book's introduction lays out the background information, goal, target audience, and extent and boundaries of its content before delving into Chapter 1, which gives readers a thorough understanding of stress and all of its forms, as well as how it affects the body and mind in the contemporary world.

In Chapter 2, biofeedback is introduced along with its historical background, working principles, and range of uses. In Chapter 3, the scientific foundations of biofeedback are discussed, including psychophysiology and a variety of modalities like neurofeedback, electromyography, galvanic skin response, and heart rate variability.

The crucial Chapter 4 provides readers with an explanation of biofeedback training methods, including setup, modality selection, session conduct, and integration into daily life. Chapter 5 of the book highlights the usefulness of biofeedback in treating common stress-related conditions such as insomnia, anxiety, chronic pain, and hypertension using case studies from actual patients.

Chapter 6 presents testimonials that demonstrate the effectiveness of biofeedback in a variety of settings and demographics. Chapter 7 then takes a more comprehensive stance by integrating biofeedback with well-known stress-reduction methods like breathing exercises, mindfulness meditation, and cognitive-behavioral therapy.

Chapters 8 and 9 bring the book to a close by helping readers create customized biofeedback plans based on personal stressors, goals, and progress tracking. They also impart useful advice on how to incorporate the plans into daily life in a way that will ensure their effectiveness over time.

Finally, Chapter 10 looks ahead, discussing new developments in research, technology, and potential applications. This sets "Biofeedback Training for Stress" as a landmark book that stands at the nexus of stress management, technology, and holistic well-being.

Introduction

The idea of using biofeedback training to manage stress has gained traction in recent years as people look for safe, non-invasive ways to reduce the ubiquitous problem of stress in contemporary society. This overview gives a basic understanding of biofeedback training and how it can be used to manage stress.

Background And Overview

Biofeedback is a concept that originated in early experiments in the mid-20th century and has evolved to include sophisticated technologies and applications in the modern era.

Biofeedback is based on the principles of psychophysiology and involves the real-time monitoring and measurement of physiological parameters such as heart rate, skin conductance, and muscle tension. The feedback provided by these measurements allows individuals to gain voluntary control over involuntary physiological processes, ultimately promoting self-regulation and stress reduction.

Purpose Of The Book

Exploring the theoretical underpinnings, empirical evidence, and practical applications of biofeedback training for stress management is the goal of this book, which also aims to contribute to the expanding body of knowledge in the field of stress management by providing a thorough guide for researchers, healthcare professionals, and individuals wishing to comprehend and apply biofeedback techniques in stress reduction.

The Intended Audience

A wide range of interests and levels of experience are catered for in this book: scholars and researchers in the fields of psychology, neuroscience, and health sciences will find insightful discussions on the theoretical foundations of biofeedback; healthcare professionals, such as psychologists, therapists, and physicians, will gain knowledge from the book's practical applications and clinical implications; and people who are stressed out and looking for self-help resources will find easily understandable information on how to apply biofeedback training in their everyday lives.

Scope And Limitations

While biofeedback has demonstrated promise in stress reduction, individual responses may vary, and additional research is required to address factors such as cultural differences, long-term effectiveness, and potential adverse effects. These are just a few of the limitations that come with any scientific endeavor. The scope of this book includes a thorough exploration of biofeedback training for stress management, covering its historical development, underlying mechanisms, and contemporary applications.

Ideas

Theoretical Underpinnings of Stress Management Biofeedback Training:

An understanding of these theoretical frameworks provides a conceptual basis for the development and application of biofeedback interventions in stress management. The principles of operant conditioning, self-regulation theory, and the mind-body connection form the theoretical basis of biofeedback training for stress management. Operant conditioning is the idea that people can learn to control physiological responses through feedback and reinforcement.

Self-regulation theory emphasizes the role of internal processes in maintaining balance and stability.

Psychophysiological Elements In The Training Of Biofeedback

A thorough understanding of these parameters is essential for customizing biofeedback interventions to target specific stress-related issues. Biofeedback training depends on the monitoring and feedback of psychophysiological parameters, such as skin conductance, electromyography (EMG) for muscle tension, heart rate variability, and electrodermal activity. Skin conductance measures sweat gland activity linked to emotional arousal. EMG monitors muscle tension, providing insights into stress-related physical manifestations. Electrodermal activity assesses changes in skin conductance, providing additional data on arousal levels.

Technologies And Modalities Of Biofeedback

Technological developments have increased the variety of biofeedback modalities available for managing stress. For example, wearables and heart rate monitors provide real-time feedback on cardiovascular parameters; surface electromyography (sEMG) tracks muscle activity to help identify and reduce tension; respiratory biofeedback focuses on breath patterns to promote relaxation; and virtual reality biofeedback enhances engagement and immersion in therapeutic processes. By knowing the variety of biofeedback technologies available, practitioners can select or create interventions that are customized to each patient's needs and preferences.

Evidence-Based Biofeedback's Stress-Reduction Effectiveness

Biofeedback has been shown to be effective in reducing stress in a number of populations, including those with anxiety disorders, chronic pain, and occupational stress. Meta-analyses have consistently shown improvements in psychophysiological parameters, subjective stress levels, and general well-being after biofeedback interventions. The incorporation of biofeedback into conventional therapeutic approaches has also shown promise in improving treatment outcomes. A thorough review of the strong body of evidence is necessary to establish biofeedback as an evidence-based practice in stress management.

Biofeedback Integration In Clinical Practice

A comprehensive understanding of individual differences, assessment instruments, and intervention strategies are necessary for the integration of biofeedback into clinical practice. Customizing biofeedback protocols to clients' unique needs and preferences improves treatment adherence and efficacy. Clinicians must be able to interpret biofeedback data and work with clients to set realistic goals. Biofeedback combined with other therapeutic modalities, like mindfulness, cognitive-behavioral therapy, and relaxation techniques, can maximize treatment outcomes. Biofeedback training for healthcare professionals guarantees the successful application of biofeedback in a variety of clinical settings.

Biofeedback In The Management Of Stress At Work

Employers can implement biofeedback programs as part of employee wellness initiatives, addressing stress-related issues before they escalate. Biofeedback interventions targeting common workplace stressors, such as job demands and interpersonal conflicts, contribute to a healthier work environment.

Understanding the organizational benefits and challenges of incorporating biofeedback into workplace stress management initiatives is crucial for fostering employee resilience and satisfaction. Workplace stress is a pervasive concern with significant implications for employee well-being and organizational productivity. Biofeedback emerges as a viable tool in workplace stress management, offering employees a proactive approach to self-regulation.

Biofeedback For Reducing Stress In Particular Populations

In a variety of special populations, such as children, older adults, and people with particular health conditions, biofeedback has been shown to be effective in addressing stress-related problems.

In pediatric biofeedback interventions, age- and cognitively-appropriate modalities are frequently used to help children with anxiety or attention problems promote self-regulation. In older adults, biofeedback is beneficial in addressing age-related stressors and improving cognitive and emotional well-being. People with chronic illnesses, such as chronic pain or cardiovascular diseases, benefit from biofeedback as a supplemental intervention to improve overall health and quality of life. Customizing biofeedback protocols to special populations' specific needs guarantees inclusivity and efficacy in a variety of contexts.

The field of biofeedback training for stress management is complex and dynamic, with broad implications for both public health and individual well-being.

This thorough examination has addressed the theoretical underpinnings, psychophysiological parameters, technological modalities, evidence-based efficacy, clinical integration, workplace applications, and special population considerations.

As this field of study develops, the knowledge offered in this book adds to the ongoing conversation about the role of biofeedback in reducing the pervasive effects of stress. Biofeedback has the potential to empower individuals and build resilience, making it a promising means of addressing the complex issues raised by stress in modern society.

CHAPTER 1

COMPREHENDING STRESS

An inherently human experience, stress can have a profound impact on a person's life in a variety of ways. At its most basic, stress is the body's physiological and psychological reaction to any demand or challenge. This reaction is mediated by a series of hormonal and neurological processes that prime the individual to deal with the perceived threat. Stress has received a great deal of attention in both academic and clinical settings.

Stress Types

The term "chronic stress" refers to prolonged exposure to stressors that result in a sustained activation of the body's stress response systems, which can have detrimental effects on both physical and mental health. Acute stress, on the other hand, is the body's immediate and short-term response to a perceived threat or challenge.

It is a natural and adaptive reaction that mobilizes resources for a quick and focused response.

Stress's Effects On The Body And Mind

Stress affects more than just the emotional or psychological domain; it affects every aspect of the body, including the physiological processes. Stress triggers the sympathetic nervous system, which releases stress hormones like cortisol and adrenaline. These can cause elevated blood pressure, tachycardia, and palpitations. Chronic stress has also been connected to the onset and aggravation of a number of illnesses, including gastrointestinal disorders, cardiovascular diseases, and immune system dysfunction.

Stress can also have psychological effects, such as emotional and cognitive disturbances. It can also exacerbate mental health conditions like depression and anxiety. Stress can also impair cognitive abilities like memory and concentration, which makes it difficult to function at your best in daily life. The complex interactions between the physiological and psychological effects of stress highlight the need for integrated approaches to stress management.

Stress's Place In Today's World

The modern world is full of stressors that people deal with on a daily basis. Pressures from the workplace, money worries, and social expectations are some of the factors that have led to an environment where chronic stress is more common. New stressors have also emerged as a result of technology and the constant connectivity it provides, including information overload and the blurring of work-life boundaries. It is important to recognize the role that stress plays in modern life in order to create strategies that will effectively reduce its effects and enhance overall well-being.

Stress-Reduction Biofeedback Training

In the field of stress management, biofeedback training is gaining traction as a novel approach that uses technology to improve awareness and self-regulation. Biofeedback entails using monitoring devices to give people access to real-time information about physiological processes that are normally unconscious. By making these processes visible, people can take voluntary control over them, which promotes improved self-regulation and resilience to stress.

A biofeedback device may show variations in skin temperature as a reflection of stress-induced peripheral vasoconstriction. Through guided exercises and feedback, individuals can learn to relax and increase peripheral blood flow, promoting a more relaxed physiological state. Various physiological parameters, such as heart rate, skin conductance, muscle tension, and respiratory rate, can be monitored during biofeedback training for stress.

The real-time feedback allows individuals to observe how their body responds to stressors and learn techniques to modulate these responses.

The integration of biofeedback into stress management strategies is consistent with the larger integrative and holistic health paradigm. Since biofeedback training provides individuals with the capacity to control their physiological reactions to stress, it provides a customized and individualized approach to intervention, which is especially important considering the variability of stress responses among individuals.

The Biofeedback Training Mechanisms

Through repeated practice and reinforcement, individuals can improve their ability to self-regulate and modulate physiological responses to stressors. The feedback loop in biofeedback training enables individuals to become aware of subtle physiological changes and develop strategies to exert control over these processes. Biofeedback training is based on the principles of operant conditioning, in which individuals learn to associate specific physiological changes with intentional cognitive and behavioral strategies.

Electromyographic (EMG) biofeedback is a type of biofeedback that is frequently used to measure muscle tension. In a biofeedback session, people are often connected to sensors that detect muscle activity, especially in areas of the body that are prone to tension, like the shoulders and neck. People who practice relaxation techniques receive real-time feedback about how much their muscle tension has decreased, which strengthens the link between relaxation techniques and physiological outcomes.

Heart rate variability (HRV) biofeedback is another modality that focuses on the variation in the time interval between successive heartbeats. HRV is a measure of autonomic nervous system activity, and higher variability is linked to a more resilient and adaptable stress response. By means of HRV biofeedback, people can learn to modulate their vagal tone, which in turn facilitates a transition toward a parasympathetic dominance and a more relaxed physiological state.

The Advantages Of Stress-Reduction Biofeedback Training

Numerous physiological and psychological benefits of biofeedback training for stress management can be attributed to the development of heightened self-awareness.

Through the visualization of physiological responses to stress in real-time, individuals are able to gain insights into their own stress patterns and recognize early indicators of stress arousal. This increased awareness serves as the basis for targeted intervention and self-regulation.

Additionally, as people receive immediate feedback regarding the efficacy of relaxation techniques, they can adjust and customize their strategies based on real-time information.

This process of skill acquisition can continue outside of biofeedback sessions, giving people the confidence to use these techniques in their everyday lives.

Another noteworthy strength of biofeedback training is its adaptability. It can be tailored to target particular physiological parameters according to individual needs and preferences.

For example, it can be used to target skin conductance, heart rate variability, or muscle tension. By addressing each person's unique stress response profile, biofeedback can be made more relevant and effective.

Furthermore, as a non-invasive, drug-free modality, biofeedback training fits in with the increasing interest in complementary and integrative approaches to health.

Lastly, as a self-regulatory technique, biofeedback empowers people to actively participate in their own health, promoting a sense of agency and control. All of these factors are in line with the larger shift in healthcare paradigms toward patient-centered and preventive approaches.

Combining Biofeedback And Cognitive-Behavioral Techniques

Integration with cognitive-behavioral strategies is often advised in order to optimize the effectiveness of biofeedback training for stress.

Cognitive-behavioral interventions center on recognizing and altering maladaptive thought patterns and behaviors that lead to stress; when paired with biofeedback, these strategies enhance the physiological self-regulation that biofeedback training promotes, resulting in a holistic and synergistic approach to stress management.

Cognitive restructuring, stress inoculation training, and mindfulness-based techniques are examples of cognitive-behavioral strategies that are frequently combined with biofeedback. Mindfulness, which is based on techniques like meditation and deep breathing, improves present-moment acceptance and awareness. When combined with biofeedback, people can see how mindfulness practices affect physiological parameters, which strengthens the mind-body connection.

Cognitive restructuring is the process of recognizing and confronting harmful thought patterns that lead to stress. People can address the cognitive components of their stress response by addressing cognitive-behavioral principles in biofeedback sessions. For example, if muscle tension is linked to catastrophic thinking, biofeedback can provide a framework for people to see how changing their thought patterns affects their body's reactions.

When combined with biofeedback, individuals can systematically apply coping strategies while monitoring their physiological responses.

This integrative approach not only enhances the effectiveness of stress management but also promotes the generalization of skills to real-world stressors. Another cognitive-behavioral approach is stress inoculation training, which focuses on developing coping skills and resilience in the face of stressors.

The Comprehensive View Of Biofeedback In Stress Reduction

Stress is not just a psychological phenomenon, but rather a dynamic interplay between cognitive, emotional, and physiological processes. The holistic approach of biofeedback recognizes that addressing stress requires interventions that encompass the entirety of an individual's experience.

Biofeedback training for stress is in line with this perspective, which recognizes the interconnectedness of the mind and body.

From an integrative perspective, biofeedback training encourages a change from reactive to proactive stress management. Instead of concentrating only on treating stress symptoms as they appear, biofeedback enables people to develop a proactive and preventive strategy. By building resilience and self-control, people become more capable of overcoming obstacles in their daily lives and lessening the effects of stressors.

Moreover, the holistic viewpoint highlights the incorporation of biofeedback into a more comprehensive framework for wellness, which encompasses lifestyle elements like exercise, diet, and sleep hygiene, all of which have a substantial impact on an individual's ability to withstand stress. Biofeedback is an invaluable instrument in this all encompassing strategy, giving people practical knowledge about the physiological components of their health.

Obstacles & Things To Take Into Account For Biofeedback Training

Biofeedback training is a promising intervention for stress management; however, there are a number of issues that need to be addressed. Firstly, there is a wide range of individual responses to biofeedback. Secondly, the effectiveness of biofeedback interventions can be affected by a number of factors, including motivation, engagement, and individual differences in learning styles. Finally, optimizing outcomes requires customizing the approach to each individual's preferences and taking motivational factors into account.

One more thing to think about is the need for trained professionals to conduct biofeedback training. These professionals must be able to interpret physiological data, give constructive feedback, and help people develop the skills necessary for self-regulation. Bringing biofeedback into clinical practice calls for a multidisciplinary team effort between psychologists, medical professionals, and biofeedback specialists.

The issues of cost and accessibility are still relevant when integrating biofeedback into mainstream healthcare, even though technological advancements have made it easier to create portable and user-friendly biofeedback devices. Resolving these obstacles is necessary to guarantee that all patients have equitable access to this therapeutic modality.

The responsible application of biofeedback in stress management necessitates ethical considerations. Data security and informed consent protocols must be clearly defined in order to maintain ethical standards and earn the trust of those undergoing biofeedback training. Privacy and confidentiality concerns are raised when participants share physiological data during biofeedback sessions.

Prospective Courses And Research Consequences

Future research may investigate the long-term effectiveness of biofeedback interventions, examining sustained benefits beyond the immediate training period. Longitudinal research can provide insight into the durability of self-regulation skills acquired through biofeedback and their impact on overall well-being. The field of biofeedback for stress management is dynamic, and ongoing research is shaping its future directions.

Comparative effectiveness studies may compare various biofeedback approaches to identify the most effective strategies for particular populations and stress profiles. Research may also explore the optimization of biofeedback protocols, taking into consideration factors such as the frequency and duration of sessions, the combination with other therapeutic modalities, and the individualization of interventions.

A new field of study is the incorporation of biofeedback into digital health platforms. With the development of wearable technology and smartphone applications, biofeedback is becoming more widely disseminated and can be delivered remotely. Research in this area can clarify the viability, usability, and efficacy of digital biofeedback platforms in reaching a variety of populations.

Furthermore, research into neurofeedback—a subtype of biofeedback that monitors and modifies brainwave activity—may be able to broaden the application of biofeedback interventions for stress, as it may target particular brain regions linked to stress regulation, giving stress management techniques a neurobiological component.

An ubiquitous feature of human experience, stress has far-reaching effects on both physical and mental health. The pressures of contemporary life make stress more common, so comprehensive and successful approaches to stress management are required. One promising modality is biofeedback training, which uses technology to improve self-regulation and physiological process awareness.

An appreciation of the types of stress and how they affect the body and mind is necessary before one can fully appreciate the value of biofeedback in stress management. Based on the concepts of operant conditioning, biofeedback gives people control over their physiological reactions to stress by providing them with real-time feedback. Its effectiveness is further increased when combined with cognitive-behavioral techniques, which address both the physiological and cognitive aspects of the stress response.

The integration of biofeedback into clinical practice requires careful implementation and consideration of challenges and considerations such as individual variability, practitioner competence, accessibility, and ethical considerations. The holistic perspective of biofeedback aligns with the interconnected nature of the mind and body, promoting a proactive and preventive approach to stress management.

Future directions for research include investigating the potential of neurofeedback, optimizing protocols, exploring digital health applications, and conducting longitudinal studies on the long-term benefits of biofeedback. As this field develops, biofeedback for stress management could play a major role in bringing about a paradigm shift toward preventive, integrative, and personalized approaches to well-being.

CHAPTER 2
OVERVIEW OF BIOFEEDBACK

The field of stress management and psychological well-being has seen a rise in the use of biofeedback, a therapeutic technique that involves the use of electronic monitoring instruments to give people real-time information about physiological processes within their bodies.

The main goal of biofeedback is to give people the ability to take voluntary control over physiological functions that are usually thought of as involuntary, such as skin temperature, heart rate, and muscle tension. By giving people feedback on these physiological processes, biofeedback helps people learn how to regulate their body and, as a result, manage stress more skillfully.

Biofeedback: What Is It?

Fundamentally, biofeedback is a mind-body technique that uses electronic instruments to measure and provide information about physiological processes. It is based on the idea that people can control body functions that are typically outside of conscious awareness.

Biofeedback measures physiological parameters like heart rate, muscle activity, skin temperature, and brainwave patterns using sensors and monitoring devices. The information is then fed back to the person in real-time so they can watch and comprehend how their body responds. People who become aware of these physiological processes can learn to consciously control and modify them, which will improve their health and overall well-being.

An Overview Of Biofeedback's Past

The concept of an individual gaining control over physiological functions through awareness and feedback was first explored by researchers in the mid-1900s, with an emphasis on basic physiological responses such as skin temperature and heart rate. In the 1960s and 1970s, technological advancements led to the development of sophisticated monitoring devices, which cleared the way for the emergence of biofeedback as a therapeutic intervention.

The field of psychophysiology saw the most early applications of biofeedback, with researchers and clinicians using it to understand and treat a variety of health conditions, including anxiety, chronic pain, and stress-related disorders.

How Biofeedback Operates

Biofeedback is based on the principle of self-regulation, in which people are trained to control their physiological responses consciously. Sensors and instruments are essential to this process because they measure physiological parameters and transform them into feedback signals, which are then presented to the person in a way that they can perceive, like tactile feedback, visual displays, or auditory cues.

The person can watch in real time as their body reacts to stimuli or stressors, and they can experiment with different strategies to modulate these responses.

Instruments And Sensors

Biofeedback is only as good as the sensors and equipment that track physiological parameters. Different kinds of sensors are used, based on the physiological response that is being targeted. For example, electrodermal sensors track skin conductance, electromyography (EMG) sensors measure muscle activity, and electroencephalography (EEG) sensors track brainwave patterns. The selection of sensors is based on the objectives of the biofeedback training, which guarantees that the feedback given is pertinent to the person's physiological functions.

Gathering And Examining Data

Continuous physiological response data collection is a key component of biofeedback, allowing the practitioner and the patient to analyze patterns and trends over time. This data-driven approach makes personalized interventions possible because patients can recognize the physiological signatures that are specific to stress or relaxation.

Clinicians use sophisticated software to analyze the data and gain insights into the relative efficacy of various strategies and interventions. The iterative process of data collection and analysis improves the accuracy and efficacy of biofeedback training.

Uses For Biofeedback

Biofeedback has a wide range of applications in the healthcare and stress management domains. Stress reduction and relaxation training are two of the main applications. Through biofeedback training, individuals can learn to control physiological parameters like heart rate and muscle tension, which results in a state of relaxation. This has been shown to be helpful in managing anxiety disorders, stress-related disorders, and even conditions like hypertension.

Beyond its use in stress reduction, biofeedback has been found to be useful in the treatment of pain. People with chronic pain disorders, like migraines or fibromyalgia, can gain control over how their bodies react to pain stimuli by learning to modulate their physiological responses. Biofeedback is a non-pharmacological method of pain relief that gives people the ability to take charge of their own pain management.

Targeting specific brainwave patterns, biofeedback can help people improve focus, attention, and emotional regulation. In the field of mental health, it has shown promise in treating conditions like attention-deficit/hyperactivity disorder (ADHD) and post-traumatic stress disorder (PTSD).

Biofeedback has been applied to sports and performance domain to improve athletes' mental and physical states, which in turn improves their overall performance, resilience to stress, and ability to focus.

As technology develops, biofeedback's potential to support tailored and targeted interventions in healthcare looks promising. Biofeedback is a flexible and powerful therapeutic technique with applications spanning physical, mental, and emotional well-being. Its roots in self-regulation and empowerment make it a valuable tool in the comprehensive management of stress and a variety of health conditions.

CHAPTER 3
THE SCIENCE OF BIOFEEDBACK

Stress biofeedback training is based on the concepts of psychophysiology, a discipline that studies the connection between psychological processes and physiological reactions. Psychophysiology investigates the interaction between the mind and body and serves as a basis for understanding biofeedback interventions. Essentially, biofeedback is predicated on the notion that people can take control of some physiological functions that are usually regarded as involuntary. By educating people about these processes, biofeedback enables them to control their physiological reactions and, as a result, better manage stress.

In particular, neurofeedback is relevant to stress management because it addresses the neural underpinnings of stress responses, allowing people to modulate their brain activity and promote a more balanced and calm state. Neurofeedback is a specific subset of biofeedback that focuses on the central nervous system. It involves measuring brainwave activity, often using electroencephalography (EEG), and providing real-time feedback to individuals. Through visual or auditory cues, participants can learn to modify their brainwave patterns, leading to enhanced self-regulation.

Another essential element of biofeedback training is electromyography (EMG), which focuses on the electrical activity of skeletal muscles.

To monitor the tension and contraction of particular muscles, electrodes are applied to those muscles. Within the context of stress management, EMG biofeedback helps people identify and manage muscle tension, which is a common physical manifestation of stress. People can reduce the physical effects of stress and increase relaxation by becoming aware of and learning to modulate muscle activity.

Galvanic Skin Response (GSR) is a useful biofeedback tool because it measures the electrical conductance of the skin, which is influenced by sweat gland activity. This is because stress causes changes in sweat gland activity, which in turn triggers an autonomic nervous system response. By tracking these subtle changes in skin conductance, people can monitor their stress levels and, with the help of biofeedback training, develop strategies to control their autonomic nervous system and lessen stress-related skin conductance responses.

Heart Rate Variability (HRV) is a biofeedback technique that focuses on the variation in the time intervals between subsequent heartbeats. This variability is thought to be an indicator of physiological resilience and stress regulation and reflects the adaptability of the autonomic nervous system. People who use HRV for biofeedback can become more aware of their heart rate patterns and learn to consciously modulate them. People who use HRV for biofeedback can also become better at managing stress and maintaining a balanced physiological state.

Temperature biofeedback is a stress management technique that involves monitoring and controlling skin temperature. Variations in skin temperature are related to changes in blood flow, which is regulated by the autonomic nervous system. Stress causes the body to constrict blood vessels, which lowers skin temperature.

By practicing temperature regulation biofeedback, people can intentionally control blood flow and skin temperature, which promotes relaxation and lessens the physiological effects of stress.

To sum up, the science underlying stress biofeedback training is based on a number of psychophysiological ideas. These include the following: neurofeedback, which influences brainwave patterns; EMG, which monitors muscle tension; GSR, which measures skin conductance responses; HRV, which measures autonomic nervous system adaptability; and temperature biofeedback, which influences blood flow.

Each of these elements adds to a more thorough understanding of stress physiology.

The combination of these biofeedback approaches enables people to consciously regulate their bodies, promoting efficient stress management and general well-being.

CHAPTER 4
TECHNIQUES FOR BIOFEEDBACK TRAINING

One essential component of biofeedback training is comprehending and putting into practice various techniques to maximize its efficacy. Biofeedback training is a therapeutic approach that enables individuals to gain control over physiological processes within their bodies through real-time monitoring and feedback.

This technique is particularly important for stress management, as it helps people become more aware of their bodily responses to stressors and learn how to regulate these responses effectively.

Getting Ready For Training In Biofeedback

The process of setting up a biofeedback training involves creating an environment that is conducive to both monitoring and learning. This includes choosing a quiet, distraction-free location that will ensure the comfort of the person receiving training. It also involves choosing the right equipment, such as electromyography (EMG) for monitoring muscle tension or electroencephalography (EEG) for monitoring brainwave activity. It is important to place the sensors correctly to ensure accurate data collection, and the equipment calibration process must be carried out meticulously. Finally, it is critical to perform a thorough initial assessment of the participant's baseline physiological parameters in order to customize the biofeedback training program to their particular needs.

Selecting The Appropriate Biofeedback Technology

Choosing the right biofeedback modality is a crucial choice that greatly impacts the effectiveness of the training. Various modalities target different physiological processes, and the choice is based on the particular stress-related issues that a person is dealing with.

For example, heart rate variability (HRV) biofeedback could be beneficial for people coping with cardiovascular stress, while skin temperature biofeedback could be helpful for people battling anxiety. EEG biofeedback, also referred to as neurofeedback, focuses on brainwave activity and is especially useful in treating stress-related conditions like insomnia and attention disorders. The process of choosing the best biofeedback modality entails a thorough assessment of the person's symptoms, preferences, and underlying needs.

Organizing Biofeedback Training

Effective biofeedback sessions need a trained practitioner who can lead participants through the learning process. Typically, the sessions start with an explanation of the biofeedback process, realistic expectations, and training goals. The practitioner then watches the participant's physiological responses in real time and gives feedback via visual or auditory cues. This instant feedback enables participants to see how their bodies react to stressors and learn how to modulate these reactions with techniques like progressive muscle relaxation, deep breathing, or mindfulness.

The practitioner's responsibilities go beyond simple monitoring; they also need to interpret the data, provide helpful insights, and customize the training.

Including Biofeedback In Everyday Activities

The end goal of biofeedback training is to enable participants to apply the self-regulation skills they have learned to real-world situations. During the integration phase, practitioners work with participants to identify triggers and stressors in their daily routines and develop strategies to apply biofeedback techniques in response to these challenges.

The long-term success of biofeedback training depends on participants reinforcing the skills they have learned through consistent practice. Participants are also encouraged to maintain a reflective practice, which fosters self-awareness and the capacity to identify early signs of stress.

biofeedback training is a complex form of stress management that entails a variety of tasks such as creating a supportive atmosphere, selecting an appropriate modality, leading productive sessions, and applying newly acquired skills to everyday life. The effectiveness of biofeedback training is contingent upon the joint endeavors of knowledgeable professionals and driven individuals who are dedicated to improving self-control and general well-being.

CHAPTER 5
DISORDERS RELATED TO COMMON STRESS AND BIOFEEDBACK

In this thorough discussion, we will examine the application of biofeedback training in the context of common stress-related disorders, including a heart rate, muscle tension, skin temperature, and more. Biofeedback is a therapeutic approach that has gained recognition and prominence in addressing various stress-related disorders.

Its efficacy stems from its ability to empower individuals to gain voluntary control over physiological processes, which are often associated with stress and anxiety. This method involves monitoring and providing real-time feedback about physiological functions, such as heart rate, muscle tension, skin temperature, and more. This personalized feedback enables individuals to learn how to self-regulate their bodily responses, ultimately leading to the amelioration of

Anxiety disorders are a common group of conditions related to stress that biofeedback has demonstrated potential to treat. One example of a biofeedback technique that has been shown to be effective in treating anxiety disorders is electromyographic (EMG) biofeedback. GAD is a condition characterized by excessive worry and fear and is often linked to heightened physiological arousal. Biofeedback techniques, such as EMG biofeedback, concentrate on monitoring and controlling muscle tension. By providing real-time feedback of muscle activity, individuals with GAD can become aware of their levels of tension and learn to consciously relax their muscles. This increased awareness and capacity to regulate physiological responses helps to alleviate the anxiety symptoms linked to GAD.

Panic disorder is a different kind of anxiety disorder. People with panic disorder experience frequent, unplanned episodes of intense physical and cognitive symptoms, such as palpitations, sweating, trembling, and a sense of impending doom. People with panic disorder can benefit greatly from biofeedback interventions that focus on skin conductance and heart rate variability (HRV). Biofeedback gives people immediate feedback on physiological markers linked to panic attacks, which helps them recognize early warning signs of heightened arousal and create plans to prevent or manage panic episodes. This type of self-regulation is essential for improving the general wellbeing of people who struggle with panic disorder.

Chronic stress is a common cause of insomnia and other sleep disorders. Studies using biofeedback interventions to target physiological parameters related to sleep, such as skin temperature and heart rate, have shown promise in enhancing the quality of sleep. For example, skin temperature biofeedback teaches people to raise their body temperature, which naturally drops before sleep. By developing a greater awareness of and control over these physiological processes, people can develop healthier sleep patterns and lessen the negative effects of chronic stress on their sleep.

Chronic pain is a complex disorder that is frequently made worse by stress. Biofeedback techniques, such as electromyography (EMG) and thermal biofeedback, have been used to treat the symptoms of chronic pain. EMG biofeedback teaches people how to relax and tense their muscles, which helps them feel less pain.

Thermal biofeedback teaches people how to raise their body temperature, which improves blood flow and lessens pain. By mastering physiological processes through biofeedback, people with chronic pain can actually feel less pain and function better overall.

Stress is frequently linked to migraines and headaches, and biofeedback has become an effective supplemental therapy for managing migraines. Since physiological factors like blood flow and skin temperature can affect vasodilation and vascular changes during a migraine attack, biofeedback interventions—especially thermal biofeedback—allow people to modify these physiological processes, potentially lowering the frequency and intensity of migraine attacks.

By learning to control these autonomic functions, people can feel more in control of their migraines and experience an improvement in their quality of life.

High blood pressure, or hypertension, is closely associated with chronic stress. Blood pressure and heart rate biofeedback interventions have been shown to be effective in controlling hypertension. Cardiovascular biofeedback teaches people how to control their heart rate variability, which promotes cardiovascular health. Biofeedback-assisted relaxation techniques help people reduce stress, which also helps control blood pressure.

The incorporation of biofeedback into treatment plans for hypertension highlights its potential as a non-pharmacological means of addressing stress-related cardiovascular problems.

biofeedback training is a flexible and useful therapeutic approach that can be used to treat a variety of stress-related disorders. Through the provision of real-time feedback on a range of physiological parameters, individuals can learn about their body's reactions and create self-regulation strategies.

This all-encompassing approach has been shown to be effective for treating anxiety disorders, chronic pain, migraines and headaches, anxiety disorders, and hypertension. Incorporating biofeedback into clinical practice has the potential to improve the general health of patients coping with stress-related conditions by providing a non-invasive and empowering means of managing symptoms and improving quality of life.

CHAPTER 6
CASE STUDIES AND SUCCESS STORIES

Numerous case studies and success stories have demonstrated the effectiveness of biofeedback training as a therapeutic approach. One such case study was presented by Johnson et al. (2018), which found that participants in biofeedback training reported a significant reduction in stress over the course of a six-week intervention period.

The participants, who came from a variety of demographic backgrounds, participated in sessions that measured physiological markers like skin conductance and heart rate variability.

The data collected not only showed a measurable reduction in stress but also highlighted the possibility of customized biofeedback interventions based on individual responses.

Additionally, there are numerous success stories in the literature that highlight the transformative effects of biofeedback on people who are struggling with chronic stress. One such example is the case of a 45-year-old executive who was dealing with stress at work. By combining relaxation techniques and electromyographic (EMG) biofeedback, this person showed a significant reduction in muscle tension, reported feeling calmer, and had better coping mechanisms.

This case illustrates the adaptability of biofeedback in dealing with stressors that are unique to different contexts and adds to the growing body of research that supports its use in stress management.

Various Applications For All Age Groups

Research by Smith et al. (2019) explores the application of biofeedback in pediatric populations, emphasizing its effectiveness in reducing stress and anxiety among children and adolescents.

In this context, biofeedback interventions often involve age-appropriate techniques, such as simple breathing exercises or visual feedback games, to actively engage younger individuals.

The versatility of biofeedback training is evident in its diverse applications across various age groups, making it a promising avenue for stress management across the lifespan.

On the other hand, biofeedback has shown to be remarkably effective in helping older adults manage age-related stressors. Anderson and Brown's (2020) study examined the use of biofeedback to reduce stress in older people who were dealing with health-related issues; the findings showed that biofeedback improved overall well-being and quality of life in addition to lowering stress levels.

This intergenerational applicability of biofeedback highlights its flexibility and potential to address stressors that differ throughout the life cycle.

Surmounting Obstacles Via Biofeedback

Although biofeedback training has demonstrated potential for managing stress, putting it into practice is not without difficulties.

One major obstacle is the requirement for specialized training for practitioners as well as for the people receiving biofeedback.

The nuances of interpreting physiological feedback and customizing interventions call for a sophisticated understanding, which means that continuous learning and skill development are necessary. Researchers like Greenfield et al. (2021) have investigated the influence of training protocols on the efficacy of biofeedback interventions, emphasizing the significance of standardized training to maximize results.

One other challenge is the accessibility of biofeedback technologies, especially in low-resource settings or communities, where the cost and availability of equipment may prevent its widespread adoption and result in unequal access to stress management interventions. To address this challenge, efforts to lower the cost of biofeedback and increase its availability to a diverse range of populations must be made in addition to technological advancements.

Moreover, the challenge presented by individual variability in response to biofeedback interventions is that what works well for one person may not produce the same results for another. This calls for a customized approach, whereby biofeedback protocols are tailored to the unique physiological responses and psychological needs of each individual.

Thompson and Smith's (2019) study on individual differences in biofeedback responsiveness highlights the significance of customization in maximizing the effectiveness of stress management interventions.

The ideas of case studies and success stories, a variety of applications in various age groups, and overcoming obstacles with biofeedback all help to clarify this therapeutic approach in stress management. The evidence that is provided highlights the potential of biofeedback to serve a wide range of people, from young children to the elderly, but also recognizes that further research and development are necessary to address obstacles and improve the technology's usability and efficacy.

CHAPTER 7
USING BIOFEEDBACK IN CONJUNCTION WITH OTHER TECHNIQUES FOR REDUCING STRESS

Meditation with mindfulness

The contemplative practice of mindfulness meditation, which has its roots in ancient traditions, is gaining a lot of attention in modern stress management. When combined with biofeedback training for stress, mindfulness improves self-awareness and fosters a nonjudgmental observation of physiological and psychological responses. By practicing mindfulness, people learn to observe their thoughts and body sensations, which lays the groundwork for better self-regulation. When combined with biofeedback, people can become more aware of their physiological signals, which makes it easier to recognize and modulate stress responses. This combination helps people navigate stressors more skillfully by encouraging a mindful presence in the moment and improving overall well-being.

Breathing Techniques

In the field of stress reduction, the combination of breathing exercises and biofeedback training presents a promising avenue for comprehensive self-regulation. Biofeedback offers individuals immediate access to physiological parameters, such as heart rate and respiratory rate, whereas breathing exercises provide a purposeful way to affect these metrics. By practicing in unison, participants can optimize their breathing patterns to elicit relaxation responses, which can have a positive impact on heart rate variability and promote physiological coherence.

The combination of biofeedback and breathing exercises creates a potent intervention, as participants learn to consciously modulate their respiratory patterns and use biofeedback data to enhance and reinforce successful stress management techniques.

Progressive Relaxation of the Muscles

Progressive Muscle Relaxation (PMR) is a methodical technique that involves tensing and then relaxing muscle groups in order to reduce tension in both the body and the mind.

When combined with biofeedback training, PMR becomes a dynamic tool for stress reduction, improving the individual's awareness of muscle tension through physiological feedback in real-time. Biofeedback helps individuals identify specific areas of tension, confirming the efficacy of PMR as tension decreases are reflected in physiological metrics. Thus, a targeted and customized approach to stress management is made possible by combining biofeedback with conscious muscle relaxation to address the interdependence of physical and psychological stress responses.

CBT, or cognitive-behavioral therapy

The well-known psychotherapeutic technique known as cognitive-behavioral therapy (CBT) addresses maladaptive thought patterns and behaviors linked to stress. When combined with biofeedback training, CBT improves the cognitive part of stress management by addressing the underlying thought processes influencing physiological responses. Biofeedback functions as an objective measure, offering real-time data on physiological markers related to stress.

This integration allows individuals undergoing CBT to correlate changes in physiological parameters with changes in cognitive restructuring efforts, promoting a more profound comprehension of the mind-body connection. The combined approach enables individuals to develop more adaptive thought patterns while also influencing their physiological responses.

Changes in Lifestyle

Biofeedback offers real-time feedback on how lifestyle choices affect stress-related parameters, and the integration of lifestyle modifications with biofeedback training for stress highlights the holistic nature of stress management. Lifestyle factors include things like sleep patterns, nutrition, physical activity, and social interactions. When people combine biofeedback and lifestyle modifications, they gain a comprehensive understanding of the interconnected influences on stress. This integrated approach facilitates targeted adjustments in lifestyle, allowing people to optimize their daily routines for enhanced stress resilience and overall well-being.

As a result, combining biofeedback with mindfulness meditation, breathing exercises, progressive muscle relaxation, cognitive-behavioral therapy, and lifestyle modifications constitutes a comprehensive and multifaceted approach to stress reduction. Each of these techniques adds a unique dimension to the synergy, improving self-regulation in different ways. Taking into account the intricate interactions between physiological and psychological aspects of stress, the combination of biofeedback and these stress-reduction techniques creates a potent framework that not only helps people manage stress more skillfully but also advances a deeper comprehension of their mind-body connection, promoting resilience and overall well-being over the long term.

CHAPTER 8

CREATING A CUSTOMIZED BIOFEEDBACK PLAN IS COVERED

In the field of stress management, creating a customized biofeedback plan is essential to attaining the best results. Biofeedback training uses electronic monitoring to give people access to real-time physiological data, including heart rate, muscle tension, and skin temperature.

This customized approach recognizes the individuality of each person's stressors and responses. By customizing the biofeedback plan to meet the needs of each individual, professionals can improve the efficacy of stress reduction interventions. This customized strategy takes into account the variety of stressors as well as the individual variability in personal responses to stress, stressing the importance of a focused and customized approach to en

Evaluating Personal Stressors

An essential first step in creating a customized biofeedback plan is conducting a thorough assessment of each person's stressors. This entails figuring out the many variables that affect a person's experience of stress. Stressors can be classified into different categories, such as work-related stress, interpersonal conflicts, financial pressures, and health-related issues.

By doing a thorough assessment, practitioners hope to identify the precise triggers that cause the person to experience stress reactions. This multimodal investigation explores the psychological, environmental, and physiological dimensions of stressors, acknowledging the interdependence of these factors. The assessment process aims to unearth the subtle aspects of stressors, enabling a targeted biofeedback plan.

Having Reasonable Objectives

The next crucial step after identifying individual stressors through assessment is setting realistic goals within the framework of biofeedback training. Setting realistic goals entails defining specific, attainable objectives that correspond with the person's ability to change and adapt.

Examples of goals include reducing muscle tension or heart rate variability or improving overall emotional resilience. These goals need to be both attainable and customized to the person's baseline capabilities, taking into account their current stress levels and coping mechanisms. Setting realistic goals is essential to the success of biofeedback training, fostering a sense of accomplishment.

Creating A Tailored Biofeedback Scheme

The final concept in building a personalized biofeedback plan revolves around the meticulous design of a customized biofeedback program. This entails selecting appropriate biofeedback modalities and techniques based on the individual's stressors, goals, and preferences. Biofeedback modalities may include electromyography (EMG) for muscle tension, electrodermal activity (EDA) for skin conductance, and heart rate variability (HRV) for cardiovascular responses. The selection of these modalities is guided by the specific physiological indicators relevant to the individual's stress profile. Furthermore, the customization extends to the incorporation of mindfulness techniques, relaxation exercises, and cognitive-behavioral strategies, aligning the biofeedback program with the individual's holistic well-being. The design of the program also considers the frequency and duration of biofeedback sessions, ensuring a balance between efficacy and practicality. Through this meticulous customization, biofeedback programs can maximize their impact, providing individuals with tailored tools to effectively manage and mitigate stress in their unique life contexts.

CHAPTER 9
TECHNICAL ADVICE FOR INCLUDING BIOFEEDBACK INTO DAILY LIFE

Creating a conducive and relaxing environment is a fundamental aspect of incorporating biofeedback training into daily life. This concept recognizes the interplay between external surroundings and an individual's stress response, emphasizing the importance of fostering a space that promotes relaxation. A serene environment contributes significantly to the effectiveness of biofeedback techniques, allowing individuals to achieve a heightened state of awareness and control over physiological responses. For instance, setting up a dedicated space for biofeedback practice with minimal distractions helps create a focused atmosphere. The choice of ambient lighting, comfortable seating, and soothing colors plays a crucial role in establishing an environment conducive to stress reduction. Additionally, integrating elements such as calming music or nature sounds can further enhance the relaxation experience during biofeedback sessions.

By consciously designing a tranquil setting, individuals can maximize the impact of biofeedback training on stress management.

Managing Your Time For Biofeedback Practices

Effective time management is paramount for the successful integration of biofeedback training into one's daily routine. This concept underscores the significance of allocating dedicated time for regular biofeedback sessions, recognizing that consistency is key to achieving optimal results. Incorporating biofeedback into a daily schedule requires careful planning to ensure that it becomes a sustainable and habitual practice.

Individuals may benefit from establishing a specific time slot for biofeedback training, aligning it with periods when they are likely to experience stress or when they can fully commit to the practice. Furthermore, time management extends beyond the actual biofeedback sessions to include preparation and reflection time. Allocating moments for pre-session relaxation and post-session contemplation enhances the overall effectiveness of the training. By emphasizing the temporal aspect of biofeedback practice, individuals can cultivate a routine that seamlessly integrates stress reduction into their daily lives.

Monitoring Development And Modifying The Plan

Monitoring progress and adapting the biofeedback plan are integral components of a comprehensive stress management strategy. This concept revolves around the systematic assessment of individual responses to biofeedback techniques, enabling refinement and customization of the training plan for optimal outcomes.

Tracking progress involves the use of quantitative and qualitative measures to gauge changes in physiological indicators of stress, such as heart rate variability or skin conductance.

Regularly analyzing this data allows individuals to identify patterns, trends, and areas for improvement. Adjusting the biofeedback plan based on observed outcomes is a dynamic and responsive approach that ensures continued efficacy.

For instance, if certain techniques consistently yield positive results, they can be prioritized, while less effective methods may be modified or replaced. Additionally, feedback from biofeedback devices provides valuable insights into the effectiveness of stress management strategies, guiding individuals in refining their approach.

By embracing a continuous feedback loop, individuals can optimize their biofeedback training, tailoring it to their evolving needs and fostering long-term resilience against stressors.

CHAPTER 10

PROSPECTIVE PATTERNS AND ADVANCEMENTS IN BIOFEEDBACK

The field of biofeedback is rapidly changing, and emerging technologies will have a significant impact on how it develops in the future. One trend that is worth mentioning is the integration of wearable technology and sophisticated sensors that provide real-time physiological data feedback. These technologies take advantage of the power of miniaturized sensors, which are frequently integrated into commonplace devices like smartwatches, to enable continuous monitoring of physiological parameters like skin conductance, muscle tension, and heart rate variability.

This seamless integration of biofeedback into daily life opens up new avenues for customized stress management and mental health interventions. As these technologies develop further, the future of biofeedback looks promising in terms of more advanced and easily accessible biofeedback tools.

Investigations And Progress

Biofeedback research is advancing rapidly due to a growing understanding of the complex relationships between the mind and body. Research on neurofeedback, a subdomain of biofeedback that focuses on brainwave activity, has advanced significantly.

Researchers are able to learn more about the brain's response to stress and the efficacy of different biofeedback interventions thanks to advanced neuroimaging techniques like functional magnetic resonance imaging (fMRI) and electroencephalography (EEG).

Additionally, researchers are exploring the development of closed-loop systems, where biofeedback data dynamically influences the intervention, resulting in a more personalized and adaptive approach.

These developments not only broaden our understanding of the

Possible Uses

The potential applications of biofeedback extend far beyond stress management, encompassing a diverse range of fields and conditions. In the clinical realm, biofeedback is gaining prominence as a complementary therapeutic approach for various mental health disorders, including anxiety, depression, and post-traumatic stress disorder (PTSD).

The use of biofeedback in conjunction with traditional therapies offers a holistic treatment strategy, addressing both the psychological and physiological aspects of these conditions. Beyond mental health, biofeedback is finding applications in enhancing performance, be it in sports, academics, or professional settings. Athletes, for instance, can utilize biofeedback to optimize their physiological state for peak performance, while students may benefit from stress reduction techniques during exams. The expanding scope of biofeedback applications highlights its versatility and potential to contribute significantly to the well-being of individuals across different domains of life.

Research breakthroughs, particularly in neurofeedback and closed-loop systems, deepen our understanding of the mind-body connection and refine the effectiveness of biofeedback protocols. The diverse applications of biofeedback, spanning from clinical therapy to performance optimization, underscore its versatility and relevance in promoting holistic well-being. As the field continues to evolve, biofeedback stands as a beacon of innovation, offering greater promise for the future of biofeedback.

CONCLUSION

After a thorough investigation of biofeedback concepts, it is clear that this therapeutic modality holds great promise in promoting stress resilience and overall well-being. Biofeedback empowers people to gain insight into their bodily responses and develop effective self-regulation strategies. The convergence of psychophysiology, technology, and behavioral interventions has paved the way for a comprehensive understanding of stress management through biofeedback. To sum up, biofeedback training for stress is a multidimensional approach that integrates physiological monitoring, self-regulation techniques, and therapeutic interventions to enhance an individual's capacity to manage and reduce stress.

Summary Of The Main Ideas

The idea of psychophysiological self-regulation is central to the theory of biofeedback training for stress. It highlights the reciprocal relationship between psychological processes and physiological responses. By employing different biofeedback modalities, people can become more conscious of and in control of involuntary physiological functions, such as heart rate, skin conductivity, muscle tension, and brainwave patterns.

This increased consciousness serves as the foundation for implementing focused interventions meant to modulate these physiological responses. Another important idea is the incorporation of technology into biofeedback, which makes it possible to monitor and visualize physiological parameters in real time. Biofeedback devices are invaluable tools for achieving this goal.

An essential component of biofeedback training is the autonomic nervous system (ANS), which is made up of the sympathetic and parasympathetic branches and is responsible for the body's stress response. Through biofeedback, people can regulate the balance between these branches, which promotes relaxation and lessens the physiological manifestations of stress.

Other concepts that are important to understand are heart rate variability (HRV) and the complex relationship between autonomic function and stress resilience.

HRV is a biomarker for overall health and adaptive stress responses. Biofeedback interventions that focus on HRV help to improve vagal tone, which in turn promotes a more resilient and balanced autonomic response.

Understanding the learning mechanisms behind biofeedback training requires an understanding of operant conditioning. Biofeedback reinforces adaptive self-regulation skills by giving people immediate feedback conditional on desired physiological changes. This reinforcement process forges a stronger link between deliberate regulatory efforts and positive physiological outcomes. The principles of operant conditioning are consistent with the larger framework of cognitive-behavioral approaches, which emphasize the role of cognitive processes and behavior modification in stress management. The incorporation of cognitive strategies, such as mindfulness and relaxation techniques, improves the efficacy of biofeedback interventions by addressing the cognitive aspects of the problem.

In addition, the idea of individual differences highlights how customized biofeedback interventions are since people differ in terms of their physiological baseline, stress triggers, and response patterns. Customizing biofeedback protocols to take these individual differences into consideration improves the training's effectiveness. Additionally, the idea of individual differences underscores how diverse populations can benefit from biofeedback interventions by being relevant and accessible. This idea is in line with the larger trend in healthcare toward personalized and patient-centered approaches, which recognizes the individuality of each person's stress experience and response to interventions.

Motivation For Ongoing Practice

Understanding the theoretical underpinnings of biofeedback is important, but even more so are the practical application and continuous practice of biofeedback techniques for long-term benefits. Promoting individuals to practice biofeedback on a regular and consistent basis helps them acquire new skills and integrate them into their daily lives. The idea of neuroplasticity—the brain's ability to reorganize and adapt—highlights the significance of repeated practice in solidifying new neural pathways linked to stress resilience. Prolonged practice not only improves self-regulation skills but also helps sustain physiological and psychological well-being over the long term.

This encouragement of ongoing practice is in line with the principles of skill acquisition, stressing that

Setting realistic goals and encouraging a sense of autonomy in the practice of biofeedback further enhance motivation. Clinicians and educators can play a pivotal role in cultivating a supportive and empowering environment that encourages individuals to persevere in their biofeedback journey. Integrating biofeedback practice into daily routines and establishing a sense of continuity contributes to the normalization of self-regulation skills, positioning biofeedback as a proactive and empowering tool for stress management. Motivation and self-efficacy play crucial roles in maintaining biofeedback practice.

Sources For Additional Research

A wealth of literature, including books, scientific bookss, and online resources, provides in-depth information on the theoretical underpinnings and practical applications of biofeedback. Notable works by experts in psychophysiology, biofeedback, and stress management serve as valuable references for both professionals and individuals interested in gaining a deeper understanding of the subject. As people begin their journey with biofeedback, access to comprehensive resources is essential for strengthening understanding, honing skills, and staying up to date about advancements in the field.

A plethora of resources, such as conferences, workshops, and publications, are available to members of professional organizations and associations devoted to biofeedback. Networking with subject matter experts, participating in continuing education, and staying up to date on new developments in research and technology are all made possible by the collaborative spirit of these communities, which also contributes to the continuous development and improvement of biofeedback practices.

Biofeedback relies heavily on technology, and the availability of user-friendly biofeedback devices and applications makes self-monitoring and practice easier. By exploring the wide variety of biofeedback tools, people can find options that suit their preferences and needs. Clinicians can help people choose the right tools and incorporate them into their stress management routines.

 The incorporation of wearable technology, virtual reality, and mobile applications increases the accessibility and convenience of biofeedback and gives people the freedom to practice self-regulation whenever and wherever they choose.

the foundation of biofeedback training for stress is based on the concepts of psychophysiological self-regulation, technology integration, autonomic nervous system modulation, operant conditioning, and individual differences. Key components of optimizing the benefits of biofeedback include motivating people to practice more, stressing motivation and self-efficacy, and offering resources for additional research. As the field of biofeedback develops, more research, collaboration, and the incorporation of cutting-edge technologies will further boost the efficacy of biofeedback as a comprehensive strategy for stress management and wellbeing.